EGG WHITES & HAM

EGG WHITES & HAM

HOW I'VE LOOKED THIS WAY FOR 15 YEARS

RYE ROBERTS

To order additional copies of this book, contact:
Xlibris Corporation
1-888-795-4274
www.Xlibris.com
Orders@Xlibris.com
47698

CONTENTS

Acknowledgment

I would like to thank several people for their contributions to this book. First, I would like to thank my dear friends, Gordon and Karry, for their inspiration to make it happen and for their professional guidance along the way. Also, thanks to Dave for his firm commitment and never-ending support. In addition, I'd like to thank Kathy, Dave, Julie, and Gordon for their editorial assistance. Last but not least, I dedicate this work to Kari and Mia for being such great cheerleaders. Thank you all so very much. I couldn't have made it happen without you!

Preface

I've always been intrigued by the Dr. Seuss book *Green Eggs and Ham©*. In this children's classic, Dr. Seuss strategically simplifies his message in a charismatic kind of way that children for decades have been able to enjoy his message. While recently reading this classic, I began to wonder, *Why couldn't it be this simple for the average adult as it pertains to their diet?* If nutrition could be made simple enough to understand, would people be able to personally relate to it to make it more effective in improving their health, in managing their weight, and in advancing their fitness levels? I believe they could. The task becomes how to simplify the complex field of nutrition so that everyone could understand it well enough to be able to effectively implement it into their lifestyle. Doing just that became the idea behind this book, *Egg Whites and Ham*.

Introduction

Quite often, I meet with people for nutritional counseling, and I am constantly amazed to see how thoroughly confused they are about nutrition and their diet. What I find myself doing is having to sit them down and try to "erase" what they thought they knew about nutrition, and literally "reinstall" the basics of what the body needs and why. These people most often have tried many different eating "schemes" or diets and just about as many times ended up right back to where they started and sometimes larger! Hence, they know what *doesn't* work.

Most often, people are what I call "sensory" eaters. This simply means they tend to eat according to how certain foods smell, sound, taste, look, or make us feel. In other words, what we eat is largely determined by some form of sensation that we can draw from it, whether it be at that current time or from memories of the past. Oftentimes, this is what we have always been taught with food. For example, remember when you were a little kid and you were fussy or maybe even got hurt? Chances are, when these times occurred, you may have been given some food item, whether it be candy or something similar, that was supposed to make you "feel" better. This starts setting up sensory fixations toward food early on. We begin to attach feelings or emotions to food and can often carry these patterns through a lifetime.

In the process of becoming "sensory" eaters, we have gotten away from paying as much attention to the real function of food for our bodies, or what I will call "functional" eating. This refers to the feeding of food to the body based on what the body "needs" in order to survive and to function properly. Can foods be eaten that serve both sensory and functional roles? Sure, and many times they do just that. Other times, however, we tend to pass up more functional foods for foods that tend to provide more emotional support rather than good functional support. This is where our diets can begin to take us downhill. It's also where many of the common health ailments begin to form. It doesn't happen overnight, but eventually, it leads to deteriorating health.

Therefore, the goal of this book is to do two main things:

1. Simply determine what the body needs from food and describe its importance.
2. Describe how the average person can adapt it for their goals.

Chapter 1

Importance of Nutrition

Excluding things like needing oxygen out of the air we breathe or a great set of genetics, we can safely say that our lifestyle has the biggest impact on how well our bodies look and function. As part of our lifestyle, nutrition is arguably the single most important factor within our control. Nutrition is a vital substance that keeps us alive. We simply cannot live without it. The food we eat provides our bodies with these necessary substances to provide energy to carry out the numerous metabolic functions that occur at any given time. This amount of "energy" is measured in units we call calories. Even during sleep, our bodies are carrying out loads of functions. And all these functions require calories; that's energy that we get from—guess where?—FOOD! This amount of energy can be figured and is often referred to as our "resting metabolic rate (RMR)" or our "basal energy expenditure (BEE)." Surprisingly, this accounts for the largest requirement of our body's daily energy needs. It represents all energy necessary to keep your heart beating, keep your lungs breathing, even keeping your body at its core body temperature. Depending on the person and their activity levels, this amount of energy (RMR or BEE) accounts from between 60-70 percent of our body's daily calorie needs.

With this being said, it makes sense for us to have a basic understanding of nutrition. Our age, activity level, health status, or future goals largely determine just how important nutrition becomes. Let me demonstrate. We can look at three main variables largely within our control that mostly influence our health and well-being. For simplicity's sake, let's look at these "variables" like pieces to a puzzle that are going to form the foundation to our program of eating right, becoming healthy, and getting our bodies in better shape. Let's imagine this program of ours to be represented as a simple triangle.

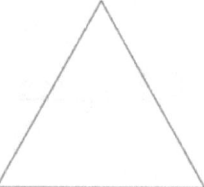

Everyone knows that a triangle consists of three sides. All three sides of the triangle need to exist and be connected in order for the structure of the triangle to stay together. For example, you've never seen a two-and-a-half-sided triangle, right? It doesn't physically exist. If it did, it wouldn't be called a triangle.

Next, let's assign each side of this triangle a variable name. Each variable will represent a factor that is within our control, that we have to work with, to make our program more complete and, in the end, can make the difference between success and failure in our quest to possess the leaner, healthier, shapelier body we're after.

Variable #1—Activity

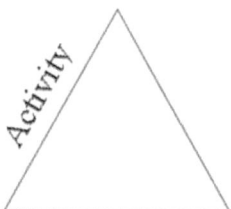

Activity requires energy, we all know that. The type, duration, and intensity of the activity determines the amount of energy required for it. As mentioned above, even during times of sleep, when there is very minimal activity, we still require a small amount of energy. On the other hand, when we partake in vigorous exercise, we understand that it takes more energy to do it. Whether we exercise or not, we generally know that it is good for us. It is something that is recommended for all of us to partake in for at least twenty to thirty minutes a day, three to four days a week. How much we do as well as how strenuous we do it determines many things about our functioning.

Variable #2—Rest and Recovery

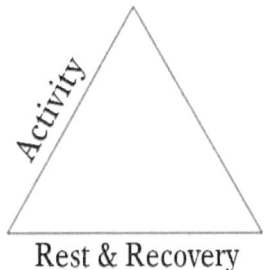

Rest & Recovery

The second lifestyle segment is rest and recovery. This is the time our body needs to recover from the daily stresses we place upon it. Whether it is physical stress from our jobs or any activity we do, or mental stress from what we go through on a daily basis, our bodies need time to rest and recover from it. How much rest and recovery we need to optimally function varies from person to person and can be saved for a topic on another day. One thing we can rest assured on (pun intended) is that our bodies need time for rest and recovery.

Variable #3—Nutrition

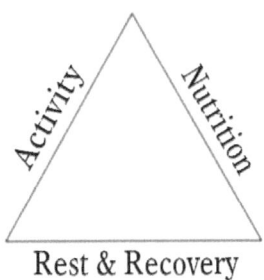

Rest & Recovery

Side three of our program lies in the scope of this book—the nutrition! Most people understand that nutrition is definitely a piece of the program, but they often don't understand the true importance that it represents. For example, depending on the person, or what their individual goals are, you will find that the nutrition factor represents between 50-75 percent of the *total* program! That's right: 50-75 percent. This may sound like a lot to contribute to the program, and many people would argue that activity has to be more prominent of a contribution, so let me break it down so that it's easier to grasp nutrition's importance here.

First, let me explain nutrition's importance to maintaining life itself in comparison to the other factors. We can live a lifetime without much exercise—and many people do—but if we cut nutrition out of the picture, we could only live for a matter of days; so it's vitally important to ensure survival. In comparison to activity and nutrition, most people get adequate rest and recovery in their every night's sleep. It is likely easier to understand nutrition's superior importance to rest. Much of the population does not get *optimal* amounts of sleep, and this is why it is a factor within our program to consider as we try to become healthier individuals.

Next, let me explain the widespread range from 50 percent all the way up to 75 percent that the nutritional factor alone represents to the program. The 50 percent importance would apply to someone who is already at a healthy normal weight, who is not dealing with any medical issues, and is looking to stay at that current point. Fifty percent of their program is going to be based within the nutrition factor alone. If we were to take a person such as this and put them strictly on a junk-food diet, chances are they would not be able to stay at a normal healthy weight and not have to deal with any medical conditions for long. Therefore, 50 percent of the program would be contained within the nutrition factor for a person of this type to stay in general good health.

What about the 75 percenters? They would be represented by most of the general population who are *not* at their optimal body weights, who are managing health conditions, or who are trying to change their body composition (this can be trying to lose fat, gain muscle, or both). Nutrition is going to play a *much, much* bigger role in the programs of these individuals. The more a person needs to change or manage, the more important nutrition becomes. With the epidemics of obesity and diabetes (type 2) the world is experiencing, it is easy to understand why most people need to emphasize a program where 75 percent is represented by the nutrition factor alone. With that being said, more emphasis also needs to be placed on an understandable way to implement healthy nutrition practices.

Chapter 2

The Six Vital Nutrients

In the last chapter, we determined just how important nutrition was to the equation to overall health. But what is nutrition exactly? This chapter breaks down what the basics are to the word we call *nutrition*. Nutrition, technically, is the science that examines the relationship between diet and health. For the purpose of this book, however, in an effort to simplify the term, nutrition will be looked at as what actually makes up the term. *Nutrition* is basically a word used to describe the combination of six vital nutrients that are required by our bodies and obtained from food and beverages we consume, to get what we need to survive and to function. In short, the six vital nutrients are protein, carbohydrates, fats, vitamins, minerals, and water.

Water:

Out of the six vital nutrients, the most important is one that many people don't even consider to be a nutrient. The reason water is so important is that our bodies are comprised of nearly 70 percent of the stuff! Basically, we are all big hairy bags of water. Water has a role in nearly *everything* that goes on within our bodies, so it literally has innumerous functions. Out of all the functions water is responsible for, three functions are so important that I want to cover them in greater detail in order to give an idea of why we should be adequately consuming it on a regular basis to properly nourish our bodies.

1.   Water's role as a transport medium.

Water is the primary means in which other nutrients are moved from point A to point B in the body. This most often occurs through the bloodstream, and guess what mostly makes up blood. That's right—water. I ask people to imagine their bloodstream much like a river. When you consider a river, how well do items move down a river when there is plenty of water in the river? Very easily, right? On the other hand, how well do items flow down a river when the river starts to dry up due to lack of water? Not so good, correct? The items start to move more sluggishly and may even tend to get backed up. The point is this: when you let yourself start to get dehydrated, your body's internal river or nutrient-transporting system starts to get a little sluggish. This sluggishness shows up as what we call our "metabolism," which I will cover in more detail a little later.

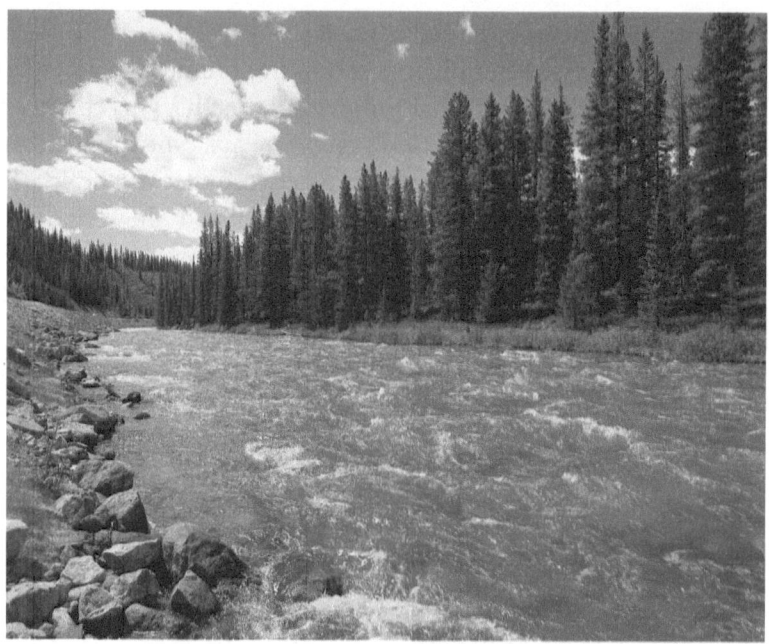

2.   Water's role as a temperature regulator.

Water is also the primary nutrient your body relies on to keep itself cool. Much like the purpose of why we put water in the radiator of our cars—water keeps the car's engine from overheating. In the human body, water does this by a process called perspiration, and happens as a result of your body heating up. This is why when we workout or just go outside on a hot day, we start to sweat. The body releases water to the surface of the skin, and as the water evaporates off the skin, it cools the body down. People don't suffer from heat exhaustion or heat stroke because the temperature approaches 100 degrees. Instead, this happens due to a lack of water—the nutrient required to regulate the body's internal temperature.

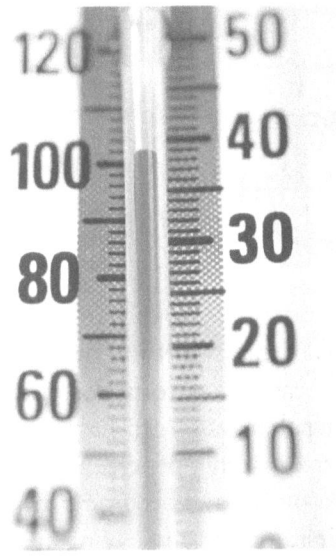

3.   Water's role as a waste manager.

To again bring in the analogy of a car, a car burns gasoline for fuel needed to operate. In the process of burning the gas for fuel, a car produces exhaust fumes as a by-product. In comparison, your body burns food for fuel. In the process of burning the food for fuel, your body produces its own by-products (called metabolic wastes) and relies on water to remove these by-products from your system. Most of these wastes are removed via the urine, but approximately 10 percent are removed through the skin. In addition, we even remove wastes (respiratory wastes) in the form of water vapor that we breathe out with each and every breath we take.

If you don't consume enough water to adequately remove these wastes from the body, they begin to accumulate within. The more the wastes accumulate, the more they act like a "deadweight" and drag down on the ever-so-popular metabolism. In comparison, it's like the car getting a sludge buildup in the engine. When it does, it just doesn't operate nearly as efficiently as it should. Much like regular tune-ups and oil changes being recommended for an automobile, regular everyday maintenance of water balance is critical and recommended for our bodies.

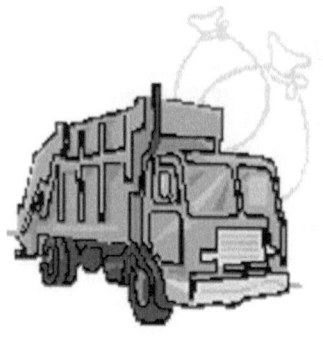 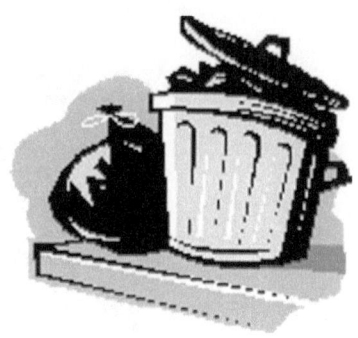

   With the explanation of these three important roles water provides to our bodies, it is hopefully an easier task to understand why we need it. To give you an idea of the impact that water can have on our bodies, consider this: At any given time, approximately 75 percent of Americans are chronically dehydrated. When we let our bodies become even mildly dehydrated, which occurs once we sense thirst, it is already having an impact. When the brain is able to sense we are thirsty, we are already mildly dehydrated. At this point, what is going on under the skin is that the nutrient-carrying river is starting to dry up and become sluggish. In addition, the metabolic wastes are starting to accumulate, further bogging down the metabolism. The overall impact is that the metabolism is going to be shut down by roughly 2-3 percent. This 2-3 percent may not sound like a lot, but at the end of a day, a 2-3 percent drop in metabolism can equate to 200-300 fewer calories per day that our bodies (and in particular, our metabolisms) are not burning because we are forcing it to operate at slower speeds due to dehydration. To put this into perspective, 200-300 calories a day would be comparable to doing 20-30 minutes of walking on a treadmill. Especially if we wanted to lose weight, wouldn't it make sense to optimize the metabolic rate by staying well hydrated? Hopefully so. This gives us yet another reason why we need to keep optimal levels of water inside our bodies.

   The next obvious question is most likely, how much water is necessary to achieve more efficient bodily operation? Many of us have heard the old adage that six to eight glasses of water a day should keep you hydrated. This is not a bad recommendation, but it doesn't take into account some very important details that can largely play a part in determining how much water intake a person is going to need. Things such as the physical size of the person (remember the body is comprised of 70 percent water, so a larger person will require more water), the activity and stress levels a person is under, as well as the temperature of the environment all influence the need for water. Therefore, a better, individualistic recommendation that I make with my clients is to take your body weight in pounds (lbs), divided by 2, to equal the number of ounces (oz) of water per day you should consume. For example, if you weigh 180 pounds, your calculations would be as follows:

$$180 \text{ lbs} \div 2 = 90 \text{ oz of water per day}$$

The above calculation would be a good recommendation for most people, most of the time. However, if it was the middle of summer and the average temperature was in the 90s and/or if you were a very active person, you will most likely need to consume more water than this to stay well hydrated. A good indicator of adequate hydration can be observed by your body's own signals. For example, your urine color can indicate your hydration status. If your urine is very light yellow in color to clear in color, it indicates you are well hydrated. On the other hand, if your urine is the color of apple juice, it is an obvious sign you are dehydrated and need to drink more water.

The above recommendations may seem to be a lot of water to consume in any given day, especially if you are not used to consuming much water. For example, ninety ounces of water is just under three-fourths of a gallon, and may seem like too much water to drink in a day. Remember, this amount of water should be consumed *throughout* the day. So if you sleep an average of eight hours a night, this leaves you sixteen hours during the day to consume the ninety ounces. Still, it may seem like too much water, and you might be thinking, "If I drank that much water, I'd be living in the bathroom." At first, it might seem that way, but one thing to remember is that our bodies are very regulatory and will adjust to the water intake. In the process of our bodies "regulating" to this new amount of water intake, we need to realize that some very important benefits will also be happening. Since our body may not be used to consuming this much water, it will have the tendency to remove the water out of the body. Here's where the benefit starts. As our body removes the excess water out of the body, guess what else the body is removing *out* along with the water—wastes! In a sense, getting adjusted to more optimal levels of water intake, your body is also going to "quick-cleanse" itself. After a few days of consistently drinking adequate amounts of water, your body will not be "releasing" as much water quite as frequently.

Several ways I get people to start drinking adequate amounts of water is to start with the following:

1. Wake up each morning and drink a full glass of water. If you take morning medicines, this is a good time to do it and have plenty of water to drink them down. It doesn't matter if you chug that glass of water down after brushing your teeth; just get it in your body first thing each day.
2. Drink a full glass of water with each meal of the day. During a meal seems to be one of the easiest times for people to drink water. Since water itself doesn't have any flavor or taste, many people aren't attracted to drinking it for this reason alone. Hence, drinking it with a meal is easier to do and realistically, is necessary; since we need water (whether in the form of tea, soda, or plain water) in the processes of digestion of the food we eat.
3. Every time you go to the bathroom to urinate, drink another glass of water, or stop by the drinking fountain (which, most of the time, is conveniently located adjacent to the restrooms) and drink eight to ten big gulps of water.
4. Always try to keep a water bottle conveniently with you at all times. The more convenient it is, the easier it is to consume. Having it within arm's reach makes it so easy to take three or four swallows, and doing so also brings in three to four ounces at a time—without even thinking about it. Besides, we all get busy in our day-to-day activities, so it's easy to see how we can overlook staying hydrated. Who wants to get up from the middle of a project at work to go visit the water fountain. Having it readily available makes it easy. Keep in mind, even if you have a desk job, a bottle of water can be conveniently kept on your desk.

These scenarios initiate a pattern that will make it easier to consume adequate amounts of water. Here's how: As you drink more water, your body is going to naturally release more water, in the form of urine. So as you drink more, you are going to urinate more. Also, as you urinate more, you will be drinking more since the third hint from above is going to have you drinking water right after using the bathroom, each and every time.

All in all, chances are going to be much greater that you will be drinking adequate amounts of water without the feeling of literally forcing yourself to drink it.

Regulating yourself to more optimal levels of water intake may only take three to four days for some, for others it might take a week; but your body will adjust to water intake. When it does, you will no longer have to remind yourself to "drink" because your body will be telling you it wants more water. At that time, it becomes an easy chore. Plus, it becomes one less nutrient to be overly concerned with. You can now direct your attention to the other vital nutrients of your diet.

The Macronutrients

The next three nutrients (proteins, carbohydrates, and fats) are collectively called the *macro*nutrients. *Macro* (meaning "many") refers to the fact that our bodies require a relatively large amount of these nutrients, because it is here where we get the energy we need to ensure survival. In addition, it is the popularity of proteins, carbohydrates, and fats that most people are familiar with nutrition as a whole. Since we *need* each of these three macronutrients, it's important to have a basic understanding of what each one is responsible for. Knowing what each of the macronutrients is responsible for in the body can help dictate how to balance them out in an effort to make the changes we're hoping to make.

Protein:

Protein in the diet is derived mainly from meat sources. We also get some of the protein in our diet from dairy (eggs, milk, yogurt, etc.), and even small amounts from foods like seeds or nuts. Protein acts as the building blocks of the body. Protein is required for structure and maintenance of many body tissues, especially muscle. For the purposes here within the scope of this book, I am mainly going to address the functions of protein as it relates to muscle tissue.

Muscle is literally a protein reservoir, and thus, proteins are the building blocks of muscle. Since muscle is metabolically active tissue within the body, muscle is directly related to metabolism. For example, the more muscle your body contains, the more active your metabolism needs to be in order to maintain that muscle. Therefore, protein is required in the diet to feed the muscles; and since muscles *are* the metabolism, we can also say that protein not only feeds the muscle, but also supports the metabolism.

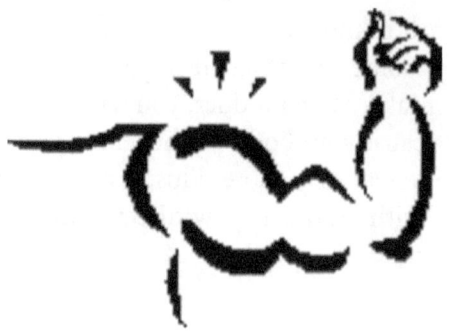

Carbohydrates:

Carbohydrates, or simply carbs, are the primary fuel source to the muscles and the metabolism. Carbs are fuel to your body, very similar to what gas is to a car engine. How well you fuel a car's engine determines how well the engine is going to run. For example, if you just bought yourself a brand-new high performance sports car, like a Ferrari, would you expect it to perform its best on the cheapest gas at the gas station, or on the premium-grade fuel available? Obviously, the better the fuel source, the better the operation, especially for a high-performance sports car. Our bodies are no different in terms of this. In fact, our bodies are much more efficient in the way they operate than the Ferrari will ever be, so optimal fuel can be ever so important to our body.

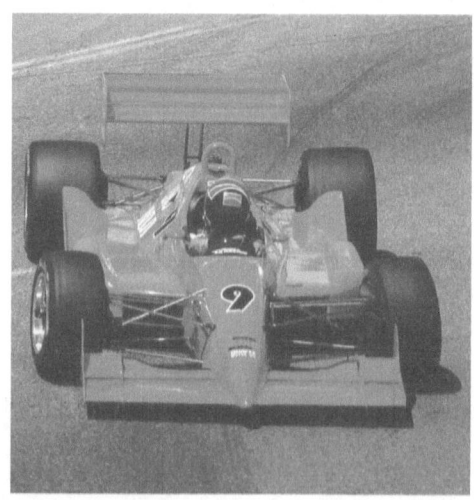

Fat:

Fat has gotten a bad reputation over the last few years, mainly stemming from the effect from what occurs when we consume too much of it. When we consistently eat too much fat in the diet, we often get fat as a result. Fat, however, provides some very vital purposes in our body. We require fat in our diets for the condition of our hair, skin, and fingernails. All these outer protective tissues rely on fat for the integrity of their cell structure. In addition, and perhaps more importantly (in terms of health and dieting), we require fat in the diet for proper hormone balance. The reason this is the case is because of the primary purpose of hormones. Hormones of any kind (and there are many inside the body) all do one common thing—regulate. Hormones regulate everything that goes on inside the body. Everything—from your hunger, to your body temperature, or your sex drive—is regulated by hormones. Therefore, having proper hormone balance in the body helps ensure proper body functioning. Because of this, I'm going to say that *indirectly*, in order to properly burn fat in our body, we need to make sure we are consuming adequate fat in our diet.

To examine this, let's say that you want to lose weight and you are jumping on board with the idea that a very low-fat diet is what you need to get the job done. The first thing you do is fill you refrigerator and cabinets with low-fat and no-fat foods of all kinds. You start to consume as low fat of a diet as you possibly can. The first thing your body is going to have to do is to tap into the stored body fat reserves and utilize this to meet its needs for functions requiring fat. At first, this appears to be a good thing and right in line with your goals, *but* remember that your body is smarter than that and is very efficient and conservative by design. Your body will only *initially* turn to the stored body fat levels, until it has time to readjust itself to function on the new very-low-fat diet that you are consuming.

Once the body has time to readjust, two very important events happen inside your body. First, your body literally tries to scrounge up any extra calories it can, and tries to convert them into—guess what?—FAT! It does this as a survival mechanism in an attempt to prepare itself for a continuing period of time, in which it may not be receiving adequate amounts of fat through the diet. The second thing that is going to happen in regulating to a very low-fat diet is your body is going to try its very best to hold on to every stitch of stored body fat extra tight. The body is trying its best to conserve what body fat it has again to prepare for the possibility of a continued future shortage in the diet.

Hopefully, neither of the above two conditions would we want to be occurring in our body. Therefore, it is just as important to be as concerned with getting *enough* fat, as it is to be getting too much. For that reason, it is recommended that you get between 20-30 percent of your daily calories from fat. This helps to meet minimum requirements for the functions that rely on fat, but yet not too much fat that it is undoubtedly going to be storing the excess as body fat.

The catch when it comes to fat intake lies in the calorie content of fat. Fat contains nine calories per gram. In comparison, both protein and carbohydrate each contain four calories per gram. Therefore, fat contains more than twice the amount of calories per gram than either protein or carbohydrate. With this being said, it is perhaps easy to understand how a little fat can go a long, long way when it is only supposed to account for 20-30 percent of the daily calorie intake.

The Micronutrients: Vitamins and Minerals

The micronutrients (vitamins and minerals) round out the six vital nutrients in the diet. Vitamins and minerals are referred to as "micro" nutrients in comparison to the macronutrients, because we require amounts much less of them in the daily diet. They can, however, be looked at as the nuts and bolts that hold the rest of the diet together. The reason is that in the many complex biochemical pathways that go on inside the body, somewhere either vitamins or minerals are required. They are also required for the body to unlock the energy hidden within any one of the macronutrients (protein, carbs, and fats). For this reason, both fruits and vegetables are highly recommended as part of a healthy diet. They both contain copious amounts of both vitamins and minerals, and should be incorporated wherever possible. Still, people often fall short on optimal vitamin and mineral intake with just food alone. This is perhaps why even the American Medical Association has come to recommend that everyone take a quality multivitamin / multimineral supplement in addition to trying to eat more fruits and vegetables.

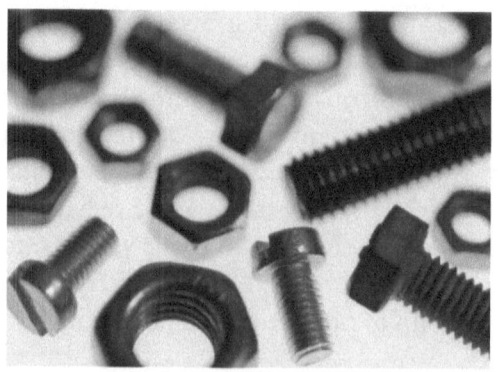

Alcohol

In summing up the six essential nutrients required by the body, I want to also spend a little time discussing another nutrient, and one that is classified as a "nonessential" nutrient. Alcohol, or more technically ethyl alcohol, is the base of many of the alcoholic beverages people consume. Whether it's a glass of wine with a nice dinner or a cold beer after work, alcohol has the ability to contribute a substantial amount of calories to the diet whenever it is consumed. One gram of alcohol will contribute seven calories. These calories, however, are referred to as "empty calories" because they hold no nutritional value to the body. Therefore, they are calories being consumed that have no real function to vital metabolic functions so they become calories your body senses as being "extra" so it metabolizes them like it would any other "extra" calories—that is, by wanting to store them. Your body will metabolize alcohol more like it would fat than it would any other nutrient.

In addition, alcohol is also a poison. That's right, it is toxic to the body; and even though it is not lethal in small doses, your body does have to detoxify the substance in order to metabolize it. This process occurs in the liver. Herein is where consuming alcohol has the ability to have a major negative impact, if consumed frequently over a long time. Being that alcohol is metabolized similar to fat, the liver can start to build up fatty residues. After years of continually metabolizing the alcohol, a "fatty liver" can begin to develop and, in later stages, can cause a condition known as cirrhosis of the liver.

For these reasons, I generally advise people to seriously limit or, better yet, try to completely avoid alcohol. It really has no place in a healthy lifestyle and is something that does have the ability to have many negative impacts to your program. If you do still wish to enjoy alcoholic beverages, do so infrequently and in moderation. Remember to consider alcohol for its relatively high calorie content and to consider these calories similar to how you would fat calories.

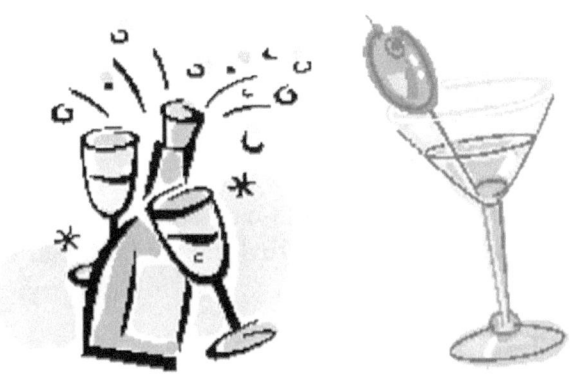

Chapter 3

Putting It All Together

In the process of putting things together in a single approach to eating right, let's start with the number one nutrient to your body—water. In order to optimize the way your metabolism is going to handle the nutrients in food, it has to begin with a well-hydrated environment. Water is going to be the agent responsible for how well nutrients get carried and delivered throughout the body. If you need to, go back to the beginning of chapter 2 to determine the minimum recommendations for your body. If you can consistently drink more water than the minimum recommendation, that is OK too. The more water you drink, the faster your results will come.

Next, we need to consider the food we eat. For the time being, forget about what you feel the best way to eat consists of, and entertain a whole new approach to feeding your body. To simplify this new approach, I want you to consider each meal of every day to consist of a three-step process.

Step 1: Choose a protein source.
Step 2: Choose a carbohydrate source relative to activity and time of day.
Step 3: Do steps 1 and 2 using low-fat foods.

Step 1 should be considered priority number 1 within each meal. Since we require protein to feed the muscle and since muscle basically *is* the metabolism, we need protein to not only feed the muscle but also to feed the metabolism. We can imagine that our muscle (and thus, our metabolism) is our internal fat-burning furnace. It would make sense, if losing body fat was our goal, to turn our fat-burning furnace on "high" every time we get the chance. By adding protein to each and every meal, it is comparable to stoking our internal metabolic fire at each and every meal. Therefore, we would want this to take top priority each and every time we eat.

Step 2 becomes second priority, and likewise, step 3 becomes third priority when you are deciding on meals. After choosing to stoke the metabolic fire in step 1, step 2 adds fuel to the fire. This determines how well the fat-burning furnace is going to function in the next few hours. If we poorly fuel the fire, we can't expect it to operate on "high" for very long. Just like the earlier example of fueling up a Ferrari, the better you fuel your metabolic fat-burning furnace, the better (and longer) it will operate in your favor.

Step 3 boils down to just making good choices in both steps 1 and 2. Sources of both protein and carbohydrate can come with varying amounts of fat. From the earlier discussion of fat pertaining to it being one of the six vital nutrients, we know that it is important to try to stay within the guidelines of a low-fat diet. This starts by first choosing low-fat foods to fill your diet with. We don't necessarily need to be consumed with choosing strictly *no*-fat foods since our bodies do require fat. The bottom line is this: if we choose most of our protein and carbohydrate foods from low-fat sources, then overall, the day's diet should likewise fall within the low-fat guideline.

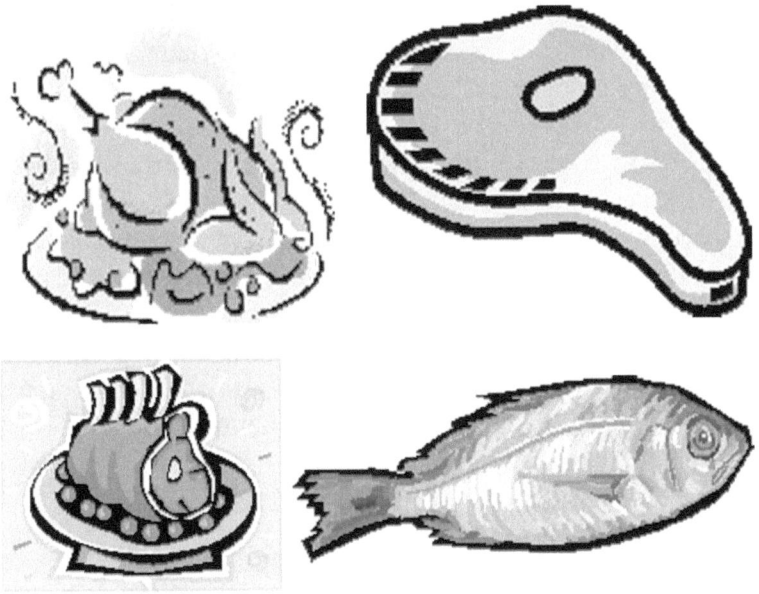

Step 1: Choosing a protein source

In choosing your protein sources, try to choose either whole meats or dairy sources, most of the time. Whole meats (like chicken, turkey, fish, beef, etc.)

contain high-quality protein. Try your best to stay away from processed meats like deli meats or lunch meats. These sources of meat are so loaded with fillers, binders, additives, and preservatives that they become inadequate sources of quality protein. These ingredients help to keep the processed meats from spoiling quite so fast, but they are not going to have any health-enhancing benefits inside your body.

Dairy sources are also quality proteins, and unless you are lactose sensitive or lactose intolerant, they usually sit well in the diets of most people. Nonetheless, dairy sources possess quality protein that is very compatible to feeding the muscle and supporting the metabolism. In considering protein sources coming from dairy foods, at the top of the list are eggs. Eggs possess high-quality protein but have received some negative attention in recent years due to cholesterol and fat content. The egg consists of two portions: the egg white and the egg yolk. The egg white is virtually 100 percent fat free easily digestible protein. Egg whites are an excellent way to provide high-quality protein needs. The egg yolk, on the other hand, is where most of the negative attention is directed. The egg yolk possesses four to five grams of fat, and another two hundred milligrams of cholesterol. The four to five grams of fat is not an outlandish amount and should not deter one from eating an occasional yolk or two. The yolk is especially rich in nutrients when you consider all the essential vitamins and minerals it contains. Eating very many yolks, however, adds up fast when you are trying to stick to a low-fat diet overall. The cholesterol content in the yolk is not as much of a concern as it once was. Several years ago, it was thought that dietary cholesterol intake may lead to high levels of health-deterring blood cholesterol levels in the human body. We now know that the body's blood cholesterol levels are more influenced by things such as genetics or saturated fat and trans-fatty acid intake rather than the actual cholesterol intake in the diet. Therefore, when it comes to eggs, we can freely use the egg white to provide our protein requirement, but we would want to limit our egg yolk consumption to one to two yolks, mainly because of the fat content contained within.

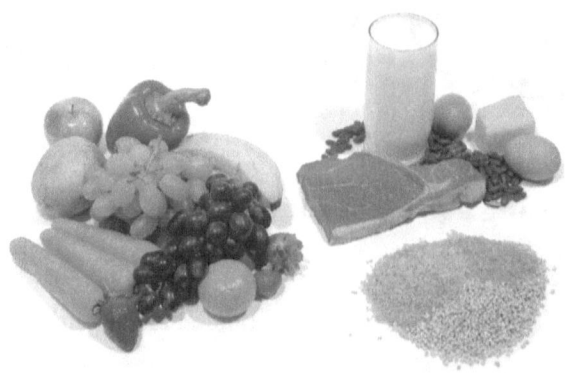

Step 2: Choose a carbohydrate source relative to activity and time of day

Carbohydrates are, without a doubt, the easiest of the six vital nutrients to find available. Most any food other than meat or any one of the oils is likely to contain some carbohydrate. Therefore, carbohydrates are literally *everywhere* in our food supply. Fitting them into the diet is all too easy, so more of the issue concerning carbohydrates lies within limiting them and choosing the right sources. The right sources are based on what the primary function carbs hold to the body—and that is to provide a fuel source. I mentioned earlier that carbs are similar to gasoline to a car's engine. The better the fuel source, the better functioning of what those fuel sources are providing energy for. To compare the quality of the fuel properties of carbs to that of gasoline, we need to look at the types of carbs they are. The low-quality carbs would be foods that contain lots of sugar (called simple sugars) and/or are highly refined or processed. Refined and processed foods have become a mainstay in the food supply of today. Any food that is no longer in the form that you would find it in nature has been processed. One way to decipher this is if a food comes in a bag or a box. If it does, then it has been processed. The more processed a food is, the less nutritional value it bears. These types of carbs are comparable to low octane-type gasoline. When we add these sources of fuel to provide energy to our fat-burning metabolism, it is similar to pouring straight gasoline onto a fire. Chances are—we all know what happens when you pour gas onto a fire—it instantly ignites. Sure it helps the fire burn, but it only burns for a very short time before it burns itself out.

The high-quality carbohydrates, while not being quite as readily available in today's food supply, are still easily accessible. These carbohydrate sources are foods we more often recognize as "health foods." Foods like fruits, vegetables, and whole grains are classic examples of high-quality carbs. They can be consumed in a form very close to how they are found in nature with very little processing. It is possible for these foods to be found in more processed states, but their true fueling value exists in the unprocessed forms. These types of body fuels would be comparable to the premium-grade fuels for your car. When we provide these sources of fuel to our metabolic furnaces, it would be comparable to throwing some wood logs onto a fire. When you do this, it isn't going to dramatically ignite the fire quite like gasoline would, but it is going to fuel the fire for a much longer period of time.

Step 3: Do steps 1 and 2 using low-fat foods

After supporting our muscles and metabolism with protein choices and then fueling them with carbohydrates, it's time to bring in step 3. Are all the foods we selected low fat? If so, the meal as a whole should also be considered a low-fat meal, meaning if we were to add up all the calories within the meal, 30 percent or less of the calories would be derived from the fat content. If you want to figure the fat content of a meal or even in a day's intake, it can be done as follows:

A. Find the total calorie count (you can use the actual food labels).
B. Count up the total amount of fat grams (again, using the food labels).
C. Take the total fat grams and multiply it by 9 (1 gram fat = 9 calories).
D. Take the number derived in step C divided by the total calorie count.
E. Multiply the number found in step D by 100, and this is the total percent that fat contributes.

Example:
Presume you added up all the calories and grams of fat (based on the serving sizes) of all the foods you ate in any certain meal. If those figures totaled 440 calories and 12 grams of fat, your calculations would look like this:

12 (grams of fat) X 9 (calories per gram) = 108 calories from fat
108 (calories from fat) ÷ 440 (total calories) = 0.245
0.245 X 100 = 24.5% of the total calories are derived from fat

Both the carbohydrate and protein selections can contribute to the fat content of the meal. For example, if your protein choice for a meal is prime rib, there is going to be a high amount of fat within. In comparison, if fish or perhaps chicken breast is your choice, very little fat is contributed from these selections. With this being the case, we would want to make most of our protein selections from the lower fat choices. To help in deciphering between high- and low-fat sources of protein, I have included the following list:

	Higher Fat Choices	**Lower Fat Choices**
Beef:	Prime rib	Sirloin
	T-bone	Fillet
	Porterhouse	Round
	Flank steak	90% or leaner hamburger
	85% lean hamburger	
	Ribs	
Chicken & Turkey:	Legs	Breast
	Thigh	
	Giblets (gizzard, liver, etc)	
Pork:	Pork chops	Loin
	Bacon	
	Ribs	
Seafood:	Salmon	Canned tuna
	Mackerel	White fish
	Sardines	Shrimp

Your carbohydrate choices vary in the ways they can contribute to the overall fat intake of a meal. Many carbohydrate choices alone, and by themselves, contain very little fat. Items such as baked potatoes or salad contain virtually no fat, but when we add on things such as butter, sour cream, or salad dressings, we bring on additional fat calories. The reason for this lies in one of the properties of fat. Fat is a very pronounced flavor carrier; so, in a sense, fat is used to liven up the flavor of whatever we are trying to bring out. Salad dressings, for example, are made with a variety of herbs and spices. When you add fat (in this case, in the form of oil, which is 100 percent fat) you are able to really amplify the flavor of those herbs and spices throughout the dressing. In addition, food choices like the baked potato are a good source of carbohydrate, but are rather bland when you eat them with nothing on them. Again, by adding a fat source, like butter or sour cream, it livens up the flavor of the baked potato. With this being understood, we need to either get used to more bland foods, learn different and more low-fat ways to flavor them, or become aware of other choices that are easier to consume without all the high-fat additions.

In an effort to give you some ideas of how you can lower the fat content with some of your carbohydrate choices, consider some of the following:

Instead of this:	Try this:
Regular salad dressings	Fat-free dressings Vinegar and lemon Salsa (makes a southwestern salad)
Baked potato with fatty condiments	Baked potato & low-fat cottage cheese Baked sweet potato (a.k.a. yam)

One important thing to add concerning fat is the differentiation between the *types* of fat. Some fats are better for you than others. Without going into a whole chapter on biochemistry, let's try to keep this as simple as we can. Consider the difference in fats as the "good" and the "not-so-good" fats. The "good" fats are those fats that are essential for body functioning and those that we have to get from our diet. These fats are less likely to be stored as body fat and are therefore more likely to be used for other more-important functions within the body. The "not-so-good" fats are the health-deterring fats that we should try to limit and, in some cases, try to avoid at all costs. They are nonessential fats, and their primary use is as a source of very dense energy, since fat contains nine calories per gram. These types of fats are preferentially stored as body fat. They have the ability to accumulate as stored body fat, only to diminish our health and wreak havoc on our physiques that we are trying so diligently to either preserve and/or improve.

The "Good" Fats

Toward the top of the list of good fats are the omega-3 fats. They have become very popular due to their health-enhancing benefits. The best-known sources of these are fish oils or the oils contained in the flaxseed. The most notable fish source of this healthy fat is salmon. As mentioned earlier, salmon is a higher-fat choice when it comes to fish; but due to its healthy fat content, it should not be overlooked in your efforts to eat a low-fat diet. These fats are good for you, so you want to consume them as part of a healthy diet.

The fat contained in the oil of the flaxseed is also a great source of the omega-3 fat. Flaxseed oil comes in a variety of forms and should all be available for purchase at your local health food stores. You can buy it as the whole seed or as the oil itself that has already been extracted from the seeds. If you choose to consume the seeds themselves, you need to make sure that you prepare them properly. The flaxseed is a small and hard seed. Consuming them whole will result in them being passed out of the system in the metabolic wastes of the body, without their healthy fats being absorbed. Therefore, you will need to grind up these whole seeds in a coffee grinder before you consume them, so your body can unlock the healthy oil contained in them. If this is the route you choose to take, you should only grind what you are going to immediately consume. Once the protective coating of the flaxseed is broken, it exposes the healthy oils. These oils are very volatile when exposed to heat, light, and air for long periods of time, and the healthy oils lose some of their benefits when this occurs. Hence, it is not recommended that you grind up a batch of the seeds and eat them over a period of days.

Flaxseed oil can also be purchased in the form of either a gel cap or as the straight oil. When searching for the oil itself, you should find it in a refrigerated section of the store. Due to the oil's volatility to heat and light, the oil should be contained in a dark-colored opaque bottle that doesn't let light penetrate through, and then stored in a refrigerated section until sold. Once you open the bottle, it is advised that you keep the lid on tight to prevent air from getting in, and then store the bottle in your home refrigerator between uses. This ensures maximum freshness and effectiveness of the healthy fats through the expiration date, which should be printed on the bottle.

Flaxseed oil can also be found in a gel cap form. Once the flaxseed oil has been encapsulated in the gel cap, it is less volatile to the environment. Still, it is a good idea to store them in the refrigerator once you have opened the bottle.

The "Not-So-Good" Fats

The "not-so-good" fats are those that we want to keep from entering our bodies as much as we can. However, they are difficult to avoid in our fat-laden food supply, and it would be nearly impossible to avoid them completely. Therefore, becoming aware of them and learning how to identify them are the first steps we can take to help diminish the health-deterring effects these fats can have.

Saturated fats are fats primarily of animal origin that are contributing factors to the declining health of many people in the world today. We have a very limited need for saturated fats since their main biological role is as a source of calories to be burned for energy. Since we all have an adequate amount of reserve body fat—that we would gladly contribute to be burned for energy—we should try to limit any more entering into our bodies. Try to make every effort to eliminate as much saturated fat from your diet as you possibly can.

Trans fats are another of the "not-so-good" fats. These fats have a very negative effect on our body's blood cholesterols—it raises the bad kind and lowers the good kind. Trans fats are chemically altered fats. They are most often recognizable from the words *hydrogenated* or *partially hydrogenated* oils. Fats are chemically altered to give them a longer shelf life, which makes them less likely to go rancid, or spoil. The biggest downfall of chemically altering fats is that it turns them into a fat our bodies can no longer use. Since our body cannot recognize the fat as something it is designed to metabolize, it preferentially is going to store it. Therefore, if improving our body composition in an effort to look and feel better is our goal, cutting the trans fats completely out of our diets makes perfect sense.

Putting All Three Steps into Action

Now that I have broken down each of the three steps, I need to describe how I recommend putting them together to work to best benefit your body. In order to do this, we need to consider the fact that each time we add food to the body, we are also adding fuel to the body, and in particular our metabolism, which, as I stated earlier, is like our fat-burning furnace. Therefore, each time we do this, we are in a sense stoking our metabolic fire to burn hotter and hotter. This is the reason I am going to suggest breaking your daily food intake up into anywhere from five to seven meals per day. However, don't think of these meals as large buffet-style meals. These meals are going to be small and nutritionally balanced. They should be designed to provide two main purposes: nourish your body for the next three to four hours, and keep you one step ahead of hunger.

Nourishing your body is about completing all three steps to effectively *feeding* the muscles (and the metabolism), *fueling* the metabolism, and doing it with low-fat foods. This is going to ensure that for the next three to four hours, your system is going to be stoked for being a calorie—and fat-burning machine. Why only three or four hours? you might ask. Because within three to four hours, your body has completely utilized whatever you ate. It doesn't matter what you eat or how much you eat. Within three to four hours after you eat, your body has metabolized it all. Once this happens, you need to restoke the metabolism: again to keep it running at full speed.

By eating nutritionally balanced meals every three to four hours, you should not have any problems with hunger pangs. Once we let ourselves get to the point where our brain is telling us we are hungry, we are entering a danger zone. When we get hungry, we become less disciplined to eat correctly. In addition, we have more of a tendency to overeat whenever we are hungry. Therefore, when hungry, the temptation to overeat and overeat on less than optimal foods deserves attention. Our best bet is to avoid these situations altogether. This is where the small meals, spaced every three to four hours apart keeps you one step ahead of hunger, and out of the potential danger zone.

An Ugly but True-to-Life Example

To illustrate the importance of the above concepts, let me sidestep here for a moment and explain the impact of *not* doing things correctly. Let's say you don't have the time or the desire to eat the five to seven small well-balanced meals a day. Therefore, you eat a meal, and it can be any meal during the day, and off you go to do other things. The next three to four hours go by in your too-busy-to-eat-right day, and you continue on with whatever you are doing. You decide to wait until you get done with your day and then go home and eat your usual large dinner meal. What just happened here is when you ate the first meal, you fed and fueled your metabolism to some degree. Then, during the next three to four hours, your body completely utilized whatever it was you ate. In doing so, your body did anywhere from one to three things with what you ate, depending on what it was and how much you ate. So let's look at these three possibilities:

1. Your body used part of what you ate to fuel whatever it was you decided to do immediately after you finished eating. Now, unless you decided to get up from eating and start doing some pretty intense activity, your immediate fuel needs were most likely more than provided for with the calorie content of your meal. Therefore, the rest of the leftover calories after providing for your immediate fuel needs went on to provide for the next step.

2. Once the immediate fuel needs were met, some, if not all, of the remaining calories filled up your secondary fuel source. This fuel

source is in a sense like a storage tank. Technically, this would be referring to your glycogen stores. Glycogen is the term used to describe the stored form of readily available carbohydrate energy. Very similar to a storage tank, there is only a limited amount of fuel that can be stored here. Once this fuel storage department is full, the remaining fuel will provide for the next step.

3. The last stop in metabolizing fuel from a meal is the reserve fuel tank. This reserve fuel tank in the body is fat. That's right, whatever fuel sources you consume that are not used for energy or used to fill up the glycogen (or readily available energy) stores goes on to be stored as fat. We have an unlimited-sized reserve fuel tank in the body. In fact, we can even grow larger, if need be, to make room for a bigger reserve fuel tank. The body is also perfectly content in keeping this fuel in the reserve fuel tank (or fat stores) until it needs it. Whether it's tomorrow or next week or next year, the body is always content to hold on to stored fuel. This goes back to how conservative our bodies are by design.

Being that this scenario is a very common situation, let's continue on with the example:

Since you decided to ignore the fact that it had been three to four hours since your last meal, your body utilized (see the above steps) all of what you ate. Your brain, which subconsciously monitors all internal activity in the body, noticed that you were running out of fuel. Hence, your brain sent a message to your body, trying to tell you a very important message. That message, if you would have known to listen, would have been saying, "hey, i'm running out of fuel here! if you don't feed me soon and this metabolism keeps running as strong as it is now, you are going to literally burn yourself up!"

Since you were too busy to take note and renourish your body, your body had to take action. Unfortunately, the action it had to take was not a desirable one. The first action your body had to take was to do all it could to uphold priority number 1—ensuring survival. Since the metabolism was still running strong from being fueled up from your last meal, your body had to find a way to turn that metabolism down in an effort to keep you from burning yourself up. To do this, your body looks to where the metabolism is most actively burning fuel, which is in the muscle tissue. (Remember, your muscle *is* the metabolism.) In an effort to turn down the metabolism, your body starts eating away at its own muscle tissue. This starts converting the fast metabolism (with lots of energy burning muscle tissue) into a smaller, more fuel efficient metabolism. However, in the process, you are also losing your hard-earned energy-burning muscle tissue at a rapid rate. This continues on until you decide to feed your body to nourish the metabolism. It is at this time that your body can stop cannibalizing your muscle tissue and start fueling the metabolism with the food you eat.

Now that you have decided to eat, is it the end of this devastating story? Not quite, so let's continue on.

After the long layover between meals, and after the loss of certain amounts of muscle tissue in the process, you finally get home and engage yourself in your dinner meal. Chances are by this time you possess a voracious appetite and could really care less what you eat as long as it is something quick. If something is not already prepared for you (perhaps by a loved one who knows all too well how you are when you get home) you are likely going to find yourself whipping something up out of convenience alone, with very little thought as to what you should be eating to effectively give your body what it needs. Therefore, you sit down (if you even take the time to sit and eat) and literally gorge yourself until you are stuffed. In the process, you have managed to eat several handfuls of chips as you were waiting for your meal to warm up. Once you had your meal you ate close to twice what you should have.

So where does this leave you in the aftermath? Well first of all, since you waited so long between meals, you built up an incredible appetite that led to you eating far too many calories at one time. On top of that, the large number of calories you consumed were most likely of low quality, high in fat (and/or sugar), and really didn't contribute anything nutritious to your body. Therefore, a small portion of the large bolus of calories quickly fills up the carbohydrate storage as glycogen, and the rest gets nestled away somewhere on your gut as body fat, where it sits and begins to accumulate through the years where one day it could possibly contribute to a severe medical condition that may (or may not) be life threatening.

This may sound like something out of a sci-fi movie, but through several years of nutritional counseling literally hundreds of people, believe me when I say that there is nothing far fetched about this story. I see it time and again. Therefore, I have to begin with each new client, just as I have with this book. I first need to stress the importance nutrition holds to the equation of health and/or fitness. Most people understand this up to a point. They know nutrition is important but didn't realize the level of importance it contributed. Secondly, I find I need to educate them on what the body really needs from food to even become or stay healthy. Then, I need to show people how to combine the nutrients throughout the day.

Getting Each Day Started the Right Way

Up to this point, I have covered the importance of nutrition as well as broken nutrition down into the six vital nutrients. We have started piecing it together by establishing the need for five to six small nutritionally balanced meals per day. This keeps our metabolisms stoked and our hunger at bay. Next, we need to continue on with how to bring in these nutrients to keep benefiting our body. The six vital nutrients need to start being brought into the body at the very first and most important meal of the day—breakfast. Chances are *your* mother, like many mothers, always stressed this to you. This was good advice and here's why. Your body has gone all night long, anywhere from six to twelve hours without any nutritional support to uphold any of the functions I discussed with the six vital nutrients. When you wake up in the morning after an overnight fast and consider the metabolism (or fat-burning fire), it resembles more of a pilot light rather than any kind of a "fire." When you don't eat breakfast, it's like saying, "I expect this little pilot light to run my whole factory (or body) until lunchtime, or whenever I decide to eat next." So how effective would this be?—not very effective at all. This helps to justify *why* we need breakfast.

Many people don't take the time for breakfast and often tell me one of two reasons: either they are simply not hungry in the morning or when they do eat breakfast, they are hungry all day. Not being hungry in the morning is nothing more than a conditioned response. It's very similar to many things, if you've done it that way for a long time, then it just becomes habit. Chances are, if these people start eating breakfast every day for a week or two and then try to go back to not eating breakfast, their bodies are going to send out all kinds of signals for them to bring in food in the morning. This is an easy habit to break and just takes a few minutes each day to correct.

The next biggest reason I hear for not eating breakfast is that breakfast makes people hungry for the rest of the day. My response: "Exactly, and that's part of why we want to eat breakfast." Breakfast is the meal that gets the body and the metabolism going. Remember, I mentioned earlier that whenever we add food to the body, we also are adding fuel to the metabolic furnace. Without breakfast, we start into our day still running in first gear. Breakfast gets us out of the starting blocks and into the fast lane for the morning.

Not only is eating the breakfast meal important, but *what* you eat for breakfast is just as important. When you look at the typical American breakfast, it consists of things like bagels, doughnuts, juice, cereal, etc. These foods contain predominately all carbohydrates with little to no protein in them. In addition, not only are they full of carbohydrates, but the carbohydrates they contain are often highly refined (processed) and/or are high in sugar. If you remember from my earlier discussion concerning carbohydrates, I mentioned that using these kinds of carbohydrates to fuel your metabolic (fat-burning) furnace is like dumping gas on a fire. They make a fire rage up but almost immediately burn out. They provide a very short lasting source of fuel. People that do this at breakfast are also those that hit that midmorning slump where they are tired and irritable and looking for some candy or a soda to give them a boost.

To correct this issue at breakfast, we can go back to the three-step approach to building a meal. Step 1 indicated including a source of protein at each and every meal. Protein is required for muscle (and metabolism) support, so adding protein to breakfast turns the pilot-like flame of the morning metabolism into a good, strong base fire. I mentioned earlier that eggs are an excellent source of protein but also fit well into the breakfast meal. As long as we limit how many egg yolks we eat, we can limit how much fat we consume in eggs. Other good sources of protein that easily fit within the breakfast meal are low-fat cottage cheese, low-fat milk, and yogurt.

Step 2 indicated adding a good source of carbohydrates to fuel the metabolic fire. By adding whole grains (like oatmeal or whole grain bread) or fruit to breakfast, you can supply fuel to the fire for hours into the morning. It's comparable to throwing logs onto a fire and knowing they will keep the fire burning. As we have seen from the example above with the typical American breakfast, we want to be sure to limit the highly processed and high-sugar sources of carbohydrates. This will keep us from going through that midmorning "crash" that comes with low blood sugar caused by our metabolic fires running out of fuel.

Third, to complete the breakfast meal, we look to step 3 of meal building. Step 3 emphasizes using low-fat foods to comprise the meal to ensure a low-fat meal as a whole. If we are conscious through our food choices in steps 1 and 2, we should have step 3 already accomplished. If all our food choices for steps 1 and 2 are very low in fat, it can leave room for us to add in an additional fat source to the breakfast meal and still fall within the guidelines of a low-fat meal. For example, we could use approximately one tablespoon of butter or peanut butter on our whole grain toast if we wanted. Even though both of these would be considered fat sources, they are natural fats, and if controlled and moderated, are still fine to fit into your diet.

One final note when it comes to the breakfast meal involves timing. Being that this meal has the largest impact on igniting the metabolism, we should strive to consume this meal within the first hour of the day. Even if you don't have an appetite upon waking up, you need to eat breakfast. Once your metabolism starts increasing through proper diet, you will find that it becomes easier to consume food first thing in the morning; but until that time, you need to be disciplined and consume the breakfast meal within the first hour of the day.

Eating for the Rest of the Day

After starting the day with a solid breakfast, a pattern begins to emerge that should be carried out for the rest of the day. Just as you did with breakfast, you repeat the three-step process to building your meals for the rest of the day. You are spacing these meals out about every three hours or so to keep the metabolic fire stoked. The only changes you make to this pattern are based on time of day and activity that exists within your day. These changes are small, and for the most part only apply to the carbohydrate nutrients.

The time of day determines the amount of carbohydrate fuel sources you should be consuming. With the breakfast meal, we can figure that you have a whole day (or several hours) of activity ahead of you, which you are going to be burning calories. Therefore, it makes sense that we can allow ourselves more carbohydrate fuel sources here versus in the evening, where we just have a few hours left in the day. It's ironic that for most people, the largest meal of the day is in the evening, or dinner meal. They consume a large amount of calories at the end of the day and then retire for the night a few hours later. On top of that, in the few hours between dinner and bedtime, they many times have one of the most inactive periods of the day, where calorie burning is slow. Whatever calories are not burned as fuel before going to sleep, will most likely be shuttled off into fat storage.

Activity is the other factor to consider when determining how many carbohydrate fuel sources we should allow ourselves. The amount and type of activity largely impacts the carbohydrate needs. If you are a very active person—say a construction worker or a lumberjack for example—you are going to be expending a lot of energy to do your daily tasks. Therefore, you are going to require more carbohydrate fuel sources all through the day than that of a more sedentary person. Even though a person is sedentary most of the day, they may have certain times when they would want to "fuel up" with more carbohydrates than usual. Activity again makes this difference. If a sedentary person is going to be exercising after work, for example, this brings in a situation where more carbohydrates could be desired. This person would want to allow themselves a few more carbohydrates than usual, to help fuel their body through the workout. Typically, the extra carbohydrates would only need to be accounted for in the meal that precedes the workout itself. Unless the individual is going to engage in very long or very strenuous activity, most often the pre-workout fueling needs can be accomplished in the pre-workout meal alone. Extreme activity can require more carbohydrates (and more overall calories) all through the day, but this is not the case concerning the average workout sessions of most people.

I've just mentioned the fact that whatever fuel sources you have not burned off by the end of the day are going to be stored as fat. This is the conservativeness that is built into your body. If there is excess energy available, it is not wasted, but rather stored, to be used at another time. So what should a person eat in the evenings to keep their bodies from accumulating body fat? You may have heard the advice, "Don't eat anything after the hours of 6:00 or 7:00 PM. Everything you eat after those times automatically gets turned into fat." That's hogwash! Your body is not on any certain time clock schedule on how it handles food and nutrients. Your activity level, as well as the rate of your metabolism on top of what you eat and how much you've eaten, determines the fate of the nutrients. If you follow the outlined three-step approach to meals, then you will likely be able to control the amount of food you eat by merely preventing your body's appetite from going crazy and leading you to overeat. Since the three steps are a balanced approach, this will likely keep you from eating the wrong types of food. Hence, when it comes to evening eating, we mainly need to be concerned about any additional fuel sources. Carbohydrates, being the *primary* fuel source to the body, and fat, being the *secondary* fuel source to the body, would need to be controlled. Protein, on the other hand, is the body's most inefficient source of fuel. In fact, just in order to convert proteins into fuel, your body has to expend roughly 25 percent of the energy contained within protein, just to make the conversion into a usable form of energy. Therefore, this makes it a very inefficient source of fuel and one that your body does not want to utilize unless it has to. Hence, protein becomes the main nutrient to gravitate toward when it comes to evening eating. Not only is it less likely to be stored as fat, but it provides the essential nutrients required for your body to repair and rebuild itself from the daily stresses placed upon it. How ironic that these processes occur at night anyway, during the restful, recuperative stages of sleep.

Dairy foods seem to be the perfect fit for evening eating. Foods such as low-fat milk or low-fat cottage cheese are excellent choices. They are low fat, low to moderate carbohydrate, and quality protein sources to help the recuperative processes that occur during sleep. In addition, they contain a type of protein called casein, which is a very slow-digesting protein, so it supplies this vital protein through several hours as we enter into the sleep cycles. Lastly, these dairy foods are good sources of the mineral calcium. Calcium helps to rebuild bone tissue, but is also a lesser know sleep aid. Calcium has a role in muscle relaxation so it can help to bring on a relaxed state, which helps initiate sleep. If you remember the old adage: "If you can't sleep at night, drink a glass of warm milk"—this is the reason. It wasn't due to fact that you were drinking *warm* milk, as it was due to the calcium contained within that it helped you get to sleep. Interesting, huh?

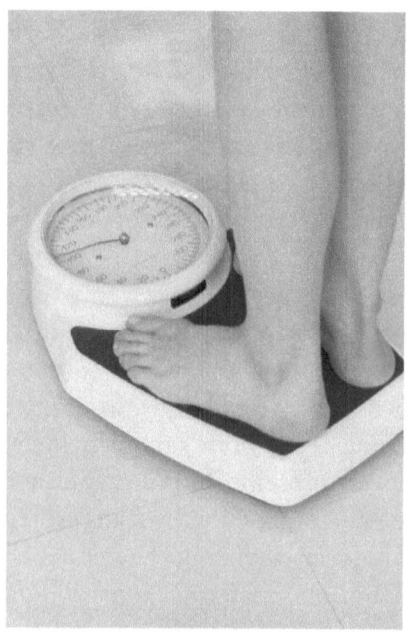
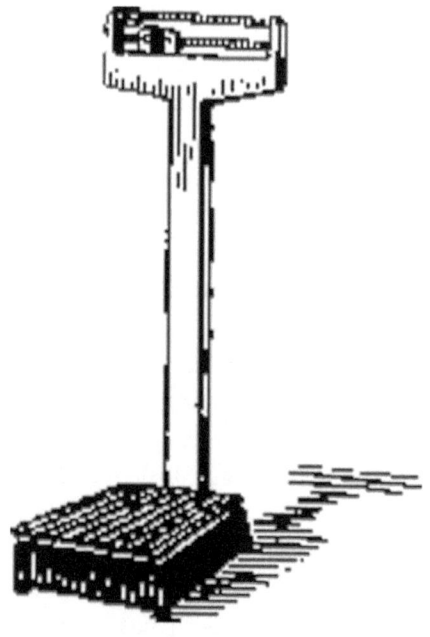

Chapter 4

The "Diet" Mentality and Weight-Loss Reality

Most people go on a "diet" in an attempt to lose weight. They understand that eating has largely contributed to getting them to where they are with their weight, so if they can make changes in their food intake, then perhaps they can start losing weight. Therein starts the search for an effective way to change their food intake to lose the unwanted weight. Most always, the typical diet attempts to target one of the three macronutrients in an effort to do one thing: produce a negative calorie balance at the end of the day, so they can lose weight. This sets up what I call the "Diet Mentality," something we have been virtually brainwashed with for years as *the* way to lose weight. Most all of the diets we have seen coming to exist through the years have been about trying to do this very thing. The concept of consuming fewer calories in a day than we burn off through our daily activities is simple energy balance, and since we derive all of our body's required energy from the three macronutrients, this makes sense to some degree. The downfall is this: it's not that simple! Our bodies are much smarter than that. If it were that simple, it would make sense that in order to lose weight *all* we would have to do is eat less. *Then*, if we wanted to lose *more* weight, *all* we would have to do is eat even less. *Then*, if we wanted to lose all the weight we wanted, *all* we would have to do is to not eat at all, and we would become the skinny, healthy individuals we want to become. Is the point clear? It's not that simple when it comes to our bodies. Sure, we can take more control over how we feed our bodies and in a sense consume fewer calories and lose some weight. *But* is this the total solution? Not quite, so let me explain.

We all know we have to eat in order to survive, so we can't go without eating. On the other hand, we understand that the human body is a very conservative and efficient machine since it was built very effectively for survival. When we simply cut our calorie intake to where it creates a negative calorie balance and continue there for an extended period of time, our body starts making adjustments internally, to adapt and become efficient in operating at this new level of calorie intake. Since it is not receiving adequate calories to maintain its current state of body composition, it immediately starts to change the body composition to become more efficient at surviving on the less-than-optimal calories we are now giving it. The result of these adjustments is the cannibalizing of the muscle tissue. With many traditional diets, this muscle wasting can account for one-half or more of the total weight a person loses. Why is so much weight lost in the form of muscle tissue rather than the more desired fat tissue? The reason is that muscle tissue is a metabolically active tissue, whereas fat is not. Fat does not require energy, or calories, for your body to maintain—muscle does. Hence, your body becomes more efficient in operating and even surviving, when it does not have to carry unnecessary amounts of energy-consuming muscle tissue.

On the flipside of this issue with the muscle tissue lies the solution for consistent, healthy weight loss. Muscle, being the metabolically active tissue that it is, is going to be your best friend, when it comes to getting your body to burn off extra calories, especially when you want those extra calories to come from the "reserve fuel tank" or stored body fat. You have to create a need for your body to use this reserve fuel, and this need comes by way of muscle. This becomes one of the main reasons I am going to suggest trying your hardest to maintain and to possibly even increase the amount of muscle in your body, if you are trying to lose fat. To begin discussing how to most effectively conserve and increase muscle tissue, we need to start by feeding the body adequately.

Consume Adequate Calories

Being that you want to lose overall body weight but wanting it to come from the stored body fat reserves and not the muscle tissue, how can this be accomplished through diet and caloric intake? First, it needs to be established that your body is getting enough calories to keep the metabolism functioning. This can be identified by calculating your BEE, or basal energy expenditure. The BEE represents the energy necessary to uphold the metabolism or the physical functioning of your body. Processes such as keeping the heart beating, respiration, digestion, etc., all require energy. The BEE is an estimation of how many calories your body is going to require for proper functioning. The calculation of BEE is performed using the following equations:

For men: BEE = 66 + (13.7 X BW) + (5 X HT) - (6.8 X Age)
For women: BEE = 655 + (9.6 X BW) + (1.7 X HT) - (4.7 X Age)

BW =   Current body weight in kilograms (take body weight in pounds
       X .45 to find your body in kilograms)
HT =   Height in centimeters (take your height in inches X 2.54 to find
       your height in centimeters)
Age = Age in years

The above calculations work for anyone who *does not* have a substantial amount of weight to lose. Once a person has a substantial amount of weight to lose, we need to make some very important adjustments in the above equations in order to find a more accurate calorie requirement for correct metabolism support. This starts by identifying a person's *desirable* body weight (DBW). By finding your DBW, we can determine if adjustments need to be made to the above BEE calculations, in order for the BEE to be accurate for any certain individual. To find your DBW, consider the following:

Men:
Allow 106 pounds for the first five feet of your height.
Add six pounds to 106 for each inch of additional height you are above five feet.
    —Example: The DBW of a five-foot, nine-inch male:
                106 + (6 X 9) = 160 lbs

Women:
Allow 100 pounds for the first five feet of your height.
Add five pounds to 100 for each inch of additional height you are above five feet.
    —Example: The DBW of a five-foot, six-inch female:
                100 + (5 X 6) = 130 lbs

Frame Size:
These equations apply to medium-framed people.
If you have a small frame, *subtract* 10 percent from the above totals.
If you have a large frame, *add* 10 percent to the above totals.

Once you calculate a person's DBW, comparing that number to your *current* body weight will determine if you need to adjust the equations for basal energy expenditure for your specific needs. Here's how: If a person's *current* body weight is less than 125 percent of the *desirable* body weight, the BEE calculations from above would be accurate. If however, a person's *current* body weight is 125 percent or more of the *desirable* body weight, then you would want to use the same BEE calculations but with an *adjusted* body weight rather than the *current* body weight.

Example #1:
    A five-foot, nine-inch man with a *small* frame weighs 138 lbs. In figuring his DBW (see above), we find his DBW to be
        DBW = 106 + (6 X 9) = 160 lbs
        DBW of 160 lbs X 10% for a small frame = 16 lbs
        DBW = 160 lbs - 16 lbs = 144 lbs

To find which of the BEE calculations that would be correct for him, multiply his *desirable* body weight by 125% (or 1.25) and compare this number to his *current* weight.
        DBW of 144 lbs X 1.25 = 180 lbs

Since his current weight of 138 lbs is lower than this calculated 125 percent of his DBW, he would need to use the BEE equation from above to find the correct number of calories for his body's metabolism.

Example #2:
    A five-foot, six-inch woman with a *large* frame weighs 222 lbs and desires to lose weight. In figuring her DBW (see above), we find her DBW to be
        DBW = 100 + (5 X 6) = 130 lbs
        DBW of 130 lbs X 10% for a large frame = 13 lbs
        DBW = 130 lbs + 13 lbs = 143 lbs

To find which of the BEE calculations would be correct for her, multiply her *desirable* body weight by 125 percent (or 1.25) and compare this number to her *current* weight.
        DBW of 143 lbs X 1.25 = 178.8 lbs

Since her current weight of 222 lbs is higher than the calculated 125 percent of her DBW, she would need to use an *adjusted* weight for her BEE equation to find the correct number of calories for her body's metabolism. In finding the *adjusted* weight for a person who is 125 percent or more of their DBW, consider the following:

$$\text{Adjusted Weight (}W_{Adj.}\text{)} = \text{(Actual weight - DBW)} \times (0.25) + \text{DBW}$$

To continue with the example of the five-foot, six-inch woman from above:

$$
\begin{aligned}
\text{Adjusted Weight (}W_{Adj.}\text{)} &= (222 - 143) \times (0.25) + 178.8 \\
&= (79) \times (0.25) + 178.8 \\
&= 198.55 \text{ lbs}
\end{aligned}
$$

The newly calculated adjusted weight ($W_{Adj.}$) becomes the new weight value to use in the original BEE equation from above. This new weight value will give an overall calorie recommendation (BEE) more conducive for the individual who weighs 125 percent or more of a desirable body weight for their height. Since the BEE is calculated in relation to body weight, it is important to consider this so not to overestimate an individual's calorie needs. By calculating the BEE, we can find the minimum number of calories we need to be consuming each day. This will help to prevent the body from decreasing the metabolic rate and thus, eating away muscle tissue.

Now that we have identified the BEE, we know the minimum calories required to keep our body functioning correctly. Next, we need to factor in the activity of our day. By doing so, we can find the total amount of calories we need to consume to give our body and our metabolism not only what it needs to function properly, but also to initiate healthy weight loss—and that is weight loss coming predominantly from stored body fat. To calculate this, I recommend multiplying the BEE by two separate activity factors. An activity factor of 1.2 would be used to represent the activities of daily living. These activities include moving around during the day doing whatever you do. An activity factor of 1.5 would be used to represent more of an active lifestyle. See below:

BEE X 1.2 = amount of calories required for an inactive day
BEE X 1.5 = amount of calories required for an active day

From here we can further emphasize our weight loss goals. We know there has to be some form of control or limitation to how many calories we can consume in order for weight loss to happen. Therefore by dropping 250-500 calories from the total amount of calories calculated when we multiplied the BEE by the two activity factors, it should give us a somewhat accurate estimation to overall calorie needs per day. I would suggest only decreasing the total calories per day by 250, so it doesn't feel like such a drastic change to your body. Keep in mind if we are optimizing the metabolic support of water in our body, we can have upward to 200-300 extra calories burned off by the metabolism alone. Couple this with a 250 calorie drop in the calculated calorie needs and we theoretically should be able to lose one pound of fat per week. I say this because we know that one pound of fat in the body is equal to 3,500 stored calories. Therefore, if we come up with a 500 calorie per day deficit, we should be able to lose one pound of fat each seven days since 500 X 7 = 3,500. Consider this:

BEE X 1.2 - 250 = minimum calories to consume on any given day
BEE X 1.5 - 250 = upper level of calories to consume on an active day

By keeping our total calorie intake in the range of calories derived from these two equations, we should also be staying within a range of calories effective to lose weight, with most of it coming from fat. The reason is that we have concerned ourselves with consuming adequate calories to keep the metabolism supported and operating effectively. Secondly, we have proportioned out our calories to be balanced with the three main macronutrients from where we get our body's energy. Lastly, we have taken into account the activity level within our day and have given ourselves a mild calorie restriction to create an energy shortage. This energy shortage should therefore be made up with energy derived by breaking down stored body fat.

The amount of calories discovered through calculating out the BEE may still need some adjustment for some individuals. If you are a sedentary to mildly active person, the calculated BEE should be very close to what calorie level you should start with. If you are a very active individual involved in three days a week or more of activity, you may need to start with 300-500 more calories than your calculated BEE. One way to tell if your BEE is correct is to monitor your weight. If you are losing more than two pounds a week for more than two consecutive weeks, you need to increase your calorie intake. Start with a 300-calorie increase and monitor your weight. If you continue to lose two or more pounds per week, add another 300 calories until your weight loss stabilizes or slows to no more than two pounds a week. Even though two or more pounds of weight loss per week may sound wonderful, we have to be careful. Don't presume that this is a good sign if it happens consistently after the initial two weeks. This can be a sign of unhealthy weight loss and a sign that your body is cannibalizing muscle tissue. Unless you are obese to morbidly obese, a weight loss of more than two pounds a week for more than two weeks in a row may need attention.

On the other hand, if you have a considerable amount of weight to lose and you start with your BEE-calculated intake without any weight loss after the first two weeks, a further decrease in calories is required. It is advisable, however, to wait for the initial two weeks to expire before decreasing your caloric intake. Your body needs some time to make the adjustments to any dietary change. Therefore, waiting the initial two weeks gives your body the necessary time it needs to fully adjust to the dietary changes. After the initial two weeks with no weight loss, start with a 300-calorie decrease and monitor your weight for a week. If no weight loss occurs after another week, decrease the calories by another 300. If you are eating correctly, you should start seeing weight loss in one, but definitely in two adjustments in calories.

Consume Ample Amounts of Protein

After calculating the BEE, you need to ensure you are eating enough protein as part of your calories. The protein needs should be met through the several small meals of the day spaced approximately every three hours. This helps to adequately feed the muscle and further support the metabolism. Your individual protein needs are going to vary considerably based on several factors. Your gender, activity level, types of activity, goals, and amount of muscle mass all influence the amount of protein you should consume. The American Dietetics Association recommends 15 percent of your calories to come from protein. Personally, if your goals are centered around losing weight, losing body fat, and maintaining or even increasing your muscle mass, I feel your protein should contribute anywhere from 25-40 percent of your total calorie intake. In some cases, where a person is incorporating vigorous weight lifting into their program, I might even advise upward to 50 percent of the calories to come from protein. To calculate the protein needs within your diet, consider the following:

1. Identify the total calorie intake for the day.   (Example 1,850 calories)
2. Identify the desired percentage of protein intake. (Example 35%)
3. Take the desired percentage of protein multiplied by the total calorie intake to find the number of calories from protein that should contribute to the total calories.   (Ex. .35 x 1,850 = 648 cal.)
4. Take the total protein calories divided by 4 (1 g. protein = 4 calories) to find the number of grams of protein required.   (Ex. 648 ÷ 4 = 162 grams)

Consume Adequate Fat

You may be inclined to keep fat intake as low as you possibly can, thinking your body will more readily tap into the stored fat reserves. This is true up to a point, but it is a very short-lived process that is only going to occur until the body begins to adapt. Once the body has the chance to make the necessary adaptations, your battle to lose unwanted body fat becomes *much, much* more difficult for you to accomplish. Therefore, we need fat in the diet to keep the body from trying to become more fat-conservative. In accomplishing this, the body will continue freeing up the stored body fat for fuel, since it is not sensing any degree of starvation or nutrient imbalance. Making sure you eat *enough* fat is just as important as making sure you don't eat *too much*. Strive to get between 20-30 percent of your total caloric intake from fat. To calculate the fat needs in your diet, consider the following:

1. Identify the total calorie intake for the day.   (Example 1,850 calories)
2. Identify the desired percentage of fat intake.   (Example 25%)
3. Take the desired percentage of fat
   multiplied by the total calorie intake
   to find the number of calories from fat
   that should contribute to the total calories.   (Ex. .25 x 1,850 = 463 cal.)
4. Take the total fat calories divided by
   9 (1 g. fat = 9 calories) to find the number
   of grams of fat required.   (Ex. 463 ÷ 9 = 51 grams)

Carbohydrates Complete the Rest

Once we have figured the desired amounts of protein and fat, carbohydrates make up the rest of the total calories. From the above example, we know we are striving for 1,850 total calories per day. Out of the 1,850 calories, 35 percent of these calories (or 162 grams) should come from protein, along with 25 percent of the calories (or 51 grams) from fat. The remaining percentage of calories (in this case 40 percent) of the calories should be made up from carbohydrates. Once we know the desired percentage, finding the amount in grams is very similar as it was for protein:

1. Take the desired percentage of carbohydrate
   multiplied by the total calorie intake
   to find the number of calories from carbohydrate

that should contribute to the total calories.   (Ex. .40 x 1850 = 740 cal.)

2. Take the total carbohydrate calories divided by
    4 (1 g. carbohydrate = 4 calories) to find the
    number of grams of carbohydrate required.   (Ex. 740 ÷ 4 = 185 grams)

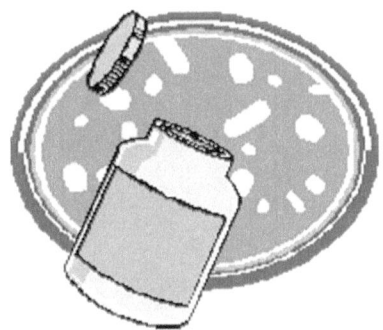

What about Supplements?

Dietary supplements have become big business. Many are advertised as if they are miracle products and all you have to do is take product X and your body is somehow going to "transform" into what you've always wanted it to become. Fact is we all know that's not going to happen. Still, nutritional supplements are a billion-dollar business.

Supplements come in many different kinds and types. Some, like vitamins and minerals, have been around for years and have some direct relevance to overall health and wellness. Others seem to be the "flavor of the day" and are nothing more than hoaxes that separate a person from their hard-earned money. They don't stand up to their promised claims and, in some cases, have resulted in multimillion dollar lawsuits. Therefore, we should always remain concerned about what we are taking. Quality of ingredients as well as in the companies that produce these products can make all the difference, even in one product to the next. If the claims made by a supplement sound too good to be true, then they probably are.

Supplements as a whole should be looked at, and therefore used, just as their name implies. Dietary supplements are designed to "supplement" the diet, meaning that your health and wellness should start with the food you eat. Supplements can then be brought into the picture to help fill any deficiencies or to make things more convenient. Used in the right way, they can make a difference and can have a role in filling in nutritional gaps in the diet.

Chapter 5

Exercise

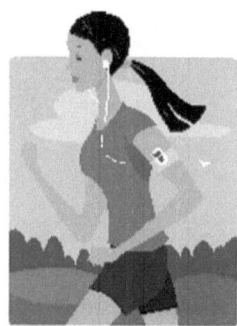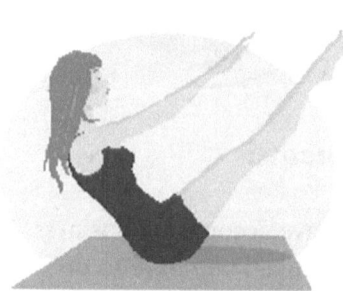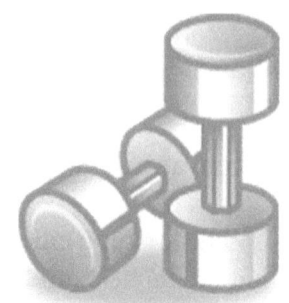

Without a doubt, a person's diet is the most important factor to a program. Diet alone will determine whether a person is going to experience success or failure in improving health or building a better body. This is why I emphasize most of your attention being placed on the way you eat. This, at least, starts you on the right path toward success. Chances are many of you have tried and failed with many things before, so let's consider another factor that will make success more in your favor. This factor is exercise. Exercise is going to contribute two main things in benefiting your program:

1. Determine the rate at which you make progress.
2. Determine *how* your body will come to *look* with the progress you make.

Being that exercise is an important factor to a healthy lifestyle, it isn't always the simplest thing to make time for. We all have busy lives without ample enough time for everything we want to do. Making time for exercise can often be met with a challenge, especially when it is not something you thoroughly enjoy doing. Try to find something you enjoy doing to make exercise part of your lifestyle. For example, if you like to golf, decide to walk the course instead of utilizing a golf cart. If time management is the concern, try doing push-ups and abdominal crunches either first thing in the morning before you shower or one of the last things in the evening before you go to bed.

For some, exercise becomes easier to commit to if there is some form of accountability involved with it. You may consider hiring a personal trainer to give you some guidance with a workout program, but just as important, to make you accountable for showing up for scheduled workouts. Likewise, finding a workout buddy to exercise with can improve your chances to get in a workout. If you would rather not depend on someone else to hold you accountable, hold yourself accountable. Set a date as your deadline to have a goal accomplished by, then set up a reward—like a vacation or a new outfit—for achieving your goal. I have even suggested for some clients to spend the money for a nice outfit they like, but in a size smaller than they currently wear to help motivate them into staying committed.

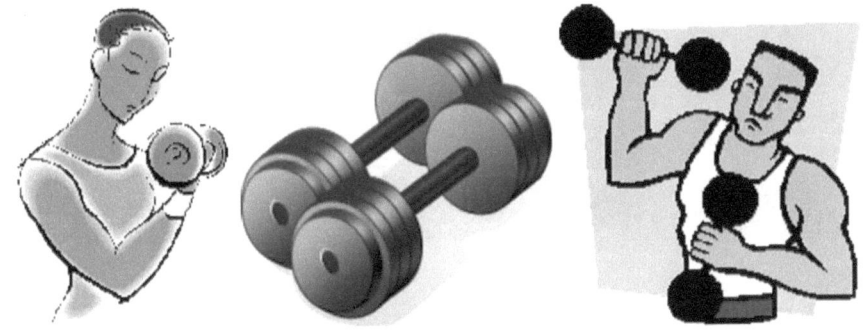

Increase Muscle with Resistance Training

Now that we have discovered how to feed the body to effectively conserve the muscle and the metabolism, what about trying to slightly increase the muscle to further enhance the metabolism? The solution resides in activity and, in particular, resistance training. Resistance training can come in different forms but perhaps the most common, is the form of weight lifting. That's right, lifting weights helps to preserve *and* build up your muscle, and, in doing so, enhances your metabolism even more. Women especially may be thinking, *But I don't want to put on muscle.* Believe me when I say, "Yes, you do!" Let me explain. Many women fear lifting weights because they think it is going to produce huge muscles, making them look like a man. This, however, is one of the biggest myths that exist in fitness, and I have to dispel this myth in nearly every female client I work with. Women, in general, do not possess high enough amounts of the natural hormones in their bodies needed to produce these huge muscles. In contrast, when women do start incorporating weight training into their program and do start to have an increase in muscle, this increase shows up as strength, firmness, tightness, and similar positive changes rather than huge muscles. Even though none of the women I work with desire to have huge muscles, I have yet to meet one that didn't want to firm and tighten up certain areas of their body. Resistance training helps to accomplish this and, in the meantime, helps to support your metabolism into becoming even more of a fat-burning machine. Therefore, I recommend spending two to three times per week resistance training for thirty minutes to an hour per session.

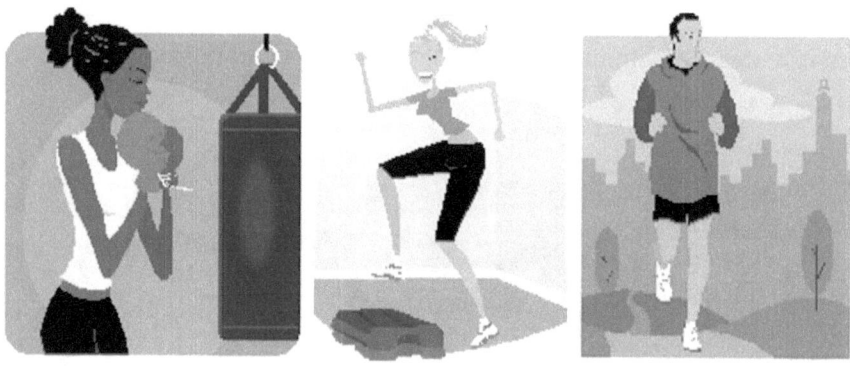

What about Cardio?

In the past, cardio, or aerobic type activity has been the predominant form of exercise recommended for losing body fat. This concept has evolved from work done at the Cooper Institute that recommended exercising at a lower intensity within a certain target heart rate zone for a period of twenty to thirty minutes. This concept emphasized your body burning a higher *percentage* of the total calories burned for this type of exercise, to be burned from fat. This is valid, but does not take into account one very important factor—that of the total calories burned and the total *amount* of fat burned as part of these calories. To simplify this consider the following:

When walking on a treadmill for an hour, a person can burn approximately 300 calories. Of these 300 calories, approximately 65 percent of the calories may come from fat. In comparison, if that same person utilized an hour lifting weights, they could realistically burn 500-600 calories, depending on the intensity, but only burn 45 percent of the calories from fat. Even though walking may burn a higher percentage of the calories from fat, doesn't mean it burns *more* fat. See below:

Walking: 300 calories X .65 = 195 fat calories burned
Lifting Weights: 500 calories X .45 = 225 fat calories burned

Since more overall calories are burned doing weight lifting, more total fat is burned despite the fact that a lower percentage of the calories burned came from fat. Therefore, the real question becomes: Are you more interested in the *percentage* of fat you burn in an exercise session, or in the total *amount* of fat burned? Your answer should be the *amount* of fat you burn.

Hopefully, this helps explain why I don't recommend you rely solely on aerobic-type activity in your goal to become healthy and build a better body. In comparison to resistance training, it doesn't burn as many overall calories or as much fat per workout session. On the other hand, I don't want to sound as if I am totally against aerobic activity either. It does have its place in a healthy lifestyle; however, it should be used to fill in the rest of the exercise equation. Aerobic activity should be incorporated into a program once resistance training is established. Adding two to three sessions of aerobic-type work on top of a program that already contains resistance training, can make it more conducive to burning fat. Therefore, if you decide to commit to more than three days a week exercising, add aerobic training on these additional days.

Body Composition

To best understand how diet and exercise is affecting our body and help to identify where and how to make necessary changes, it is truly helpful to know a person's body composition. Our bodies can be observed as a combination of two different types of tissues that make up our body composition. Body composition is both fat mass and fat-free mass, and each is often expressed as a percentage of the body weight of an individual. Fat mass is just as the name indicates—*fat*, or more technically, adipose tissue. We all know what fat mass is: it's the tissue responsible for us not being able to fit into our jeans anymore. It's the tissue that hangs over our belts. It's also the tissue that is largely responsible for the epidemic of obesity and other health conditions in the world today. The fat that resides in our bodies, however, isn't always a bad tissue. We all need body fat in order to survive. Body fat is actually a stored form of energy, and we rely on this energy each and every day—whether we realize it or not. Fat also provides functions such as insulating heat to the body and cushioning the organs to protect them from damage. Therefore, we have to have body fat in order to survive, but when we accumulate too much of it, it starts to have an adverse affect and become a detriment to our health.

In comparison to fat mass, fat-free mass is most all other tissues in the body. This tissue accounts for everything from bone, muscle, organs, and water. In other words, if it's *not* fat, then it can be grouped into the tissue known as fat-free mass. For most people, the fat-free mass accounts for most of the body weight when a person weighs themselves on a scale. However, in some cases of obesity, a person's fat mass can outweigh their fat-free mass. Again, this is not a healthy measure, and one in need of improvement.

Conclusion

Nutrition as a whole is not an easily understood topic. However, for all practical purposes and to be best suited for most people, nutrition can be simplified into understanding the basics. Basic nutrition is what any diet is built upon. This doesn't change. The six vital nutrients covered in this book still come up first for consideration in *any* diet. These nutrients provide us with energy to function and the necessary components to ensure survival. It's literally impossible to get away from this. Therefore, having a basic understanding of what each of these nutrients are as well as what role they play in the body is important to know. Likewise, having a good guide to fit them into the diet is going to help prevent many of the deficiencies in most of today's "fad diets." Once we can gain a basic understanding of what our bodies need out of food and why it's important, we can then start the journey toward better health and wellness. This journey can then more easily become a lifestyle and be directed toward specific goals such as weight loss, muscle toning, or improved performance. I encourage you to really embrace the concepts outlined in this book in guiding you toward better health and wellness. Happy journeys!

EGG WHITES & HAM

HOW I'VE LOOKED THIS WAY FOR 15 YEARS

The "Rye Roberts" Story

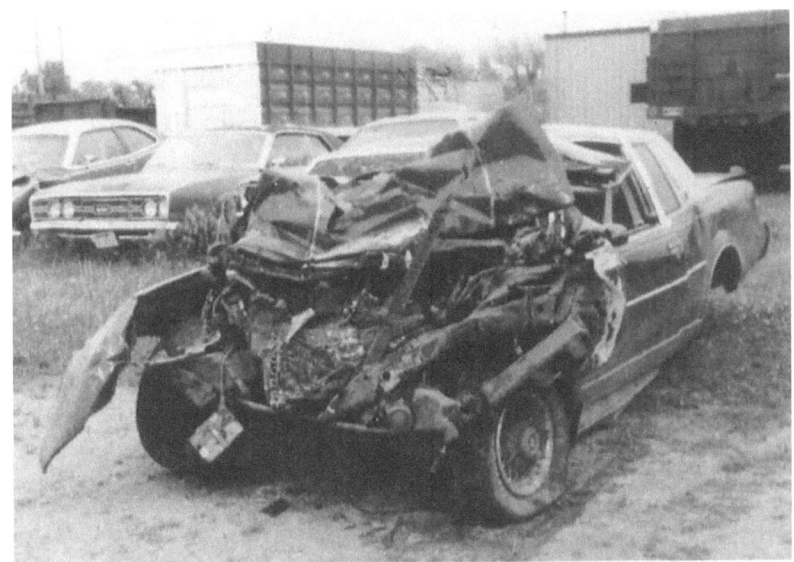

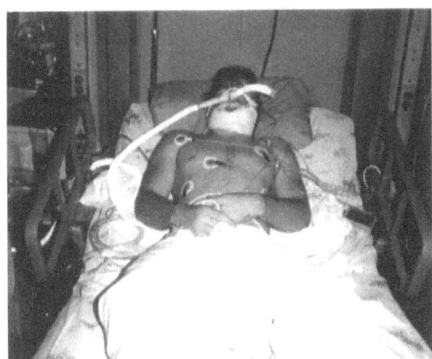 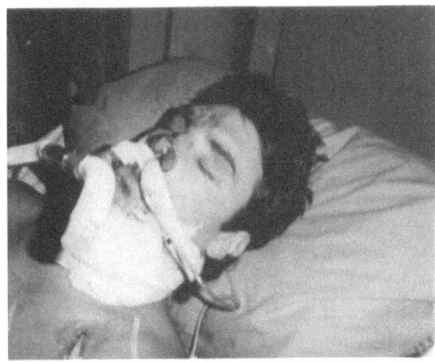

My life was not always about eating right and taking care of my body. I received a "blessing in disguise" that changed this however, and started me on a course that has lasted almost 20 years. This "blessing" came by way of an automobile accident that happened the day before I was to graduate from high school. Prior to that day, I was a typical youth from a blue-collar upbringing. My early years were filled with the growing-up phases that most any kid goes through. During high school I played sports, hung out with friends, and like any other teenager, contemplated what profession to choose when I grew up.

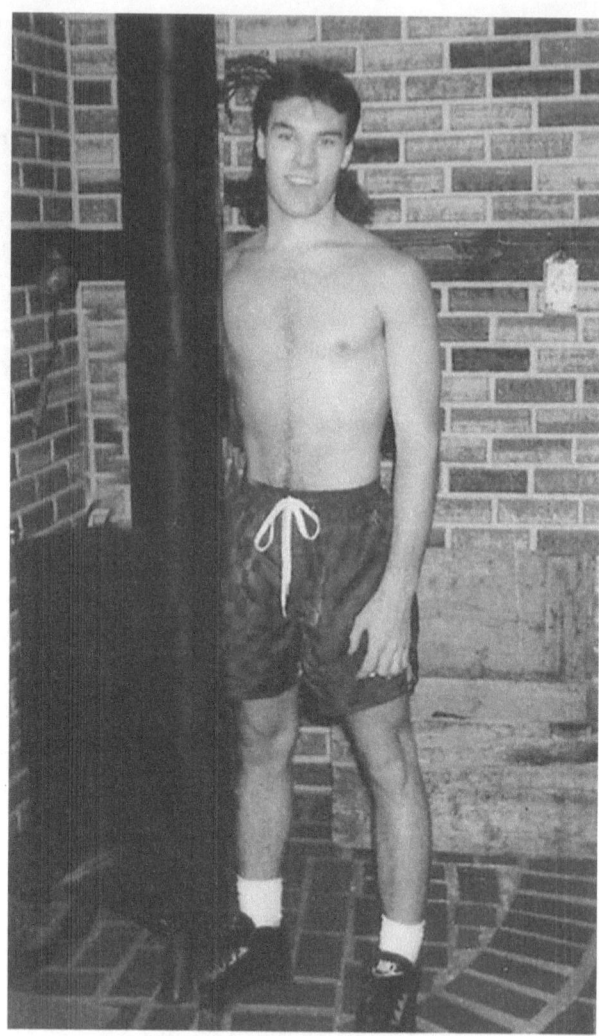

The auto accident literally took my world by storm. I recovered from it just fine, but in the process had lost 25 pounds and most of the athletic physique I had acquired from playing sports and working out. For an in-shape 18 year old, this was pretty devastating. Obviously, I lived through this and was able to go on to college and start my journey towards the rest of my life. The first couple years of a typical college life led to my gaining back the weight I had lost from the accident, plus some. In comparison through, I didn't quite look like I did when I was active in sports.

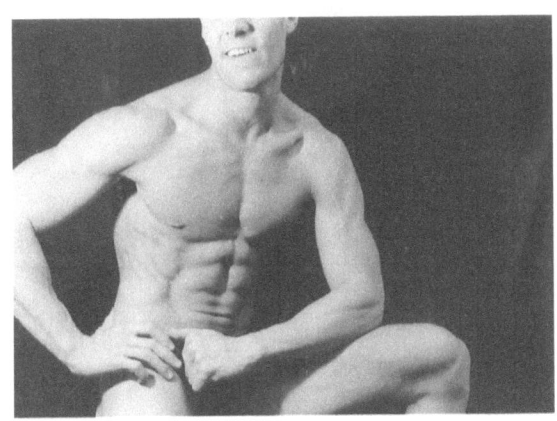
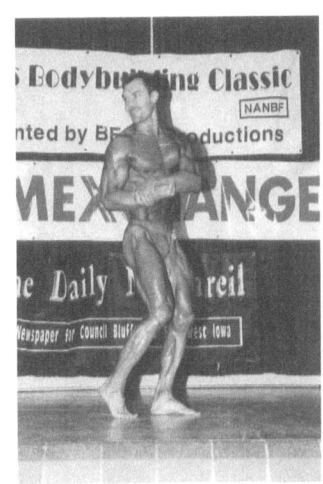

During my junior year of college, I decided enough was enough. I vowed to take control of my health, my weight, and my physique. I started working out and trying to eat better even on my college budget. In the process I was going to learn all I could to make better choices. My main source of inspiration became the countless fitness magazines that lined the supermarket checkout counters. I figured this, on top of my college course work for a Pre-Med major, would be a good start to building the shapely body I had committed to achieve. This however, brought me to finding both the value and the confusion of nutrition.

It was ever so obvious that nutrition held a HUGE role in accomplishing my goals. If I was going to learn how to lose body fat and both tone and shape muscle, I was going to have to get this nutrition thing down. I tried several different "diets" and numerous supplements with only limited success. One thing I did discover was that there are many ways to do it wrong.

I graduated from college and did not get accepted into medical school. Instead of just sitting idle and re-applying the following year, I decided to make the leap into the field of nutrition. I entered graduate school and spent the next two and a half years earning my Master's Degree in Nutritional Science and Dietetics. I then became qualified as a Registered Dietitian so I could legally practice in the nutrition field. This education proved effective in learning the scientific principles in understanding the details of nutrition. Meanwhile, putting the education to work in my personal body quest also proved to be effective. I was able to get my body into shape and carry single digit body fat percentages year-round ever since.

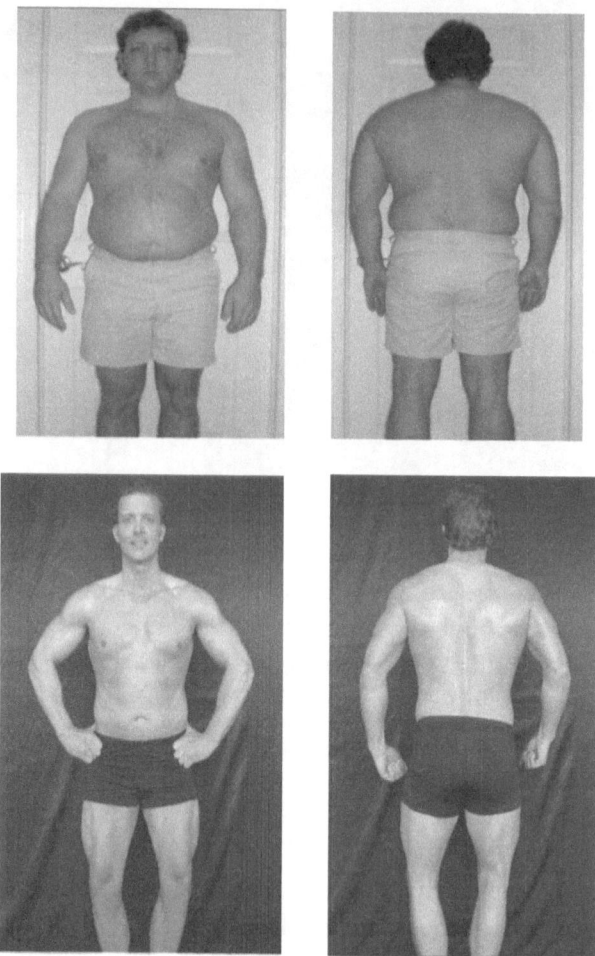

Gordon's transformation

This brings me to the scope of this book. I have put together more than 10 years of practice into simple principles that have been tried and tested by countless numbers of my clients. As shown in the above photos, Gordon Whitten came to me weighing 224 pounds, with a waistline of 38 inches, and a body fat percentage of 18.5. After 12 weeks utilizing my nutrition principals, (along with a structured resistance training program) he now weighs 186 pounds, has a waistline of 33 inches, and a body fat percentage of 9.5. Gordon is just one example of how my easy-to-understand approach to nutrition can have life changing results. My goal is to break down the scientific stuff into simple principles that the average person can understand and utilize for themselves. I bring this to you in an easy to read book that will guide you step-by-step in the process of using nutrition to improve your body. I hope you enjoy it.

My "Top 10" Personal Recommendations

1. Drink copious amounts of water.
2. Eat adequate calories.
3. Eat ample amounts of protein.
4. Eat enough fat while focusing especially on omega-3 fats.
5. Alter carbohydrate intake relative to time of day and activity.
6. Eat meals frequently.
7. Incorporate resistance training two to three times per week.
8. Lose weight slowly.
9. Limit alcohol intake.
10. Utilize food first, before supplements.

Rye Roberts, MS, RD, LMNT, can be contacted for individual consultations or public appearances through the following contacts:

e-mail:	*ryeroberts@cox.net*
Phone:	(402) 660-1251
Web site:	*www.xlibris.com/EggWhites&Ham.html*
Address:	Rye's Fitness & Nutrition, Inc.
	7301 South 93rd Street
	Omaha, NE 68128

Testimonials

"Rye is a great nutritionist because he understands not only the science of nutrition but the emotion and reasoning involved in why eating healthy can be so difficult. While working with Rye, he explained everything in simple, easy to understand terms which I was able to apply to my own life.

Rye helped me to learn exactly how my diet can affect my body and how nutrition can be every bit as important (if not more) than exercise.

Thanks Rye!"

Dave Fichter

"I pretty much grew up on pizza, fast food, sweets, and soda. I was an athlete in high school and college, so sports always kept me from realizing how poor my diet really was. I never really understood the ramifications of eating so badly. Then, when I finished college and settled into my career, I put on 40 pounds almost overnight. I found myself in my mid 20's out of shape, out of breath, and overweight. I finally got sick of it and went on a "diet." I tried numerous approaches and was able to lose weight for periods of time, but I never kept it off. I was up and down, up and down. As I got into my 30's, I found it harder and harder to have these swings. I was looking for something that could help me change once and for all but did not know what to do. I needed a better plan, and I needed accountability. I adopted Rye's diet principles that include six small meals per day packed with high quality protein. I lift three days per week and do cardio some of the off days. This plan got me looking and feeling the best I ever have. At 36, I can honestly say I am in the best shape of my life. Rye has truly been key to getting me through this major lifestyle change. I am very appreciative of all he has done, what he has taught me, and for the friendship that has been built along the way. I am never going back."

Gordon Whitten, Omaha, NE

"After having my second child, I wanted to get back into pre-baby shape. I followed the simple nutrition guidelines outlined in this book, coupled with a basic resistance training and cardio exercise program, and I was back to my pre-pregnancy weight in no time. It was so easy to follow I've continued to incorporate the principles into my everyday lifestyle. It's been simple to maintain, and I look and feel better now than I ever have."

Kathy Rygg, age 34

"Everyone has a different reason for making changes in their life. For me, it was after my last birthday that I realized it was time to do something for *me*. I consider it fate that I found Rye Roberts. Rye put health, nutrition, exercise—everything—into perspective and helped me realize I could and should do this for myself. Rye leads without pushing and teaches without preaching; all while making goals feel attainable. There is nothing in his nutritional wisdom that isn't completely doable. It all makes sense now, but it took someone passionate about this knowledge to show me the way. It doesn't matter where you are in your life; I am a believer that Rye's knowledge and expertise in nutrition can help you improve your life. I am learning to embrace the knowledge that Rye has given me. He is a motivator, mentor, and friend."

Julie Huff

"When I met Rye I had tried every diet out there with nothing to show for it but frustration. At 5'6" weighing 257 pounds and the age of 52, I did not think I would ever learn what I needed in order to live a better life. I was wrong. I have learned that nutrition is a big part of what you have to do. I never thought I could eat so much and feel so great about myself.

Nutrition is a big part of my life now along with exercise and making sure I get the rest I need. I feel great about living this new life style."

Vicki Clingerman

Index